THRUSH

EVERYTHING ABOUT THRUSH
TREATMENTS THAT YOU DIDN'T KNOW

DR. J. WALLER

Contents

INTRODUCTION

Candida species most commonly, Candida albicans cause the fungal infection known as thrush, usually referred to as oropharyngeal candidiasis. White, creamy lesions on the tongue, inner cheeks, and other oral mucosa areas are often the outcome of this ailment, which mostly affects the mouth and throat. Although the yeast Candida is a normal part of the oral and digestive system, an overabundance of it can cause thrush, particularly in people who are at risk due to other reasons or compromised immune systems.

Creamy white lesions that may resemble cottage cheese are indicative of thrush, which can cause discomfort, burning feelings, and difficulty swallowing. Although it can afflict people at any age, newborns, elderly people, and people with weakened immune systems are more likely to experience it.

For an accurate diagnosis and course of treatment, it is imperative to comprehend the causes, symptoms, and risk factors related to thrush. Thrush is managed in part by taking antifungal drugs and treating underlying issues. Reducing the incidence of thrush also requires preventive steps and good oral hygiene habits.

CHAPTER ONE

Description of Thrush

Thrush, also known as oropharyngeal candidiasis, is a fungal infection that develops in the mouth and throat due to an overabundance of the species Candida, most often Candida albicans. One kind of yeast that typically lives in the mouth and gastrointestinal system without harming people is called candida. But in other cases, such when the immune system is compromised, when antibiotics are taken, or when other circumstances throw off the delicate balance of bacteria, Candida can grow and cause thrush.

Important Points:

Causative Agent: Thrush is caused by species of Candida, mainly Candida albicans.

Location: On the tongue, inner cheeks, roof of the mouth, and other oral mucosa regions, thrush appears as creamy white, cottage cheese-like lesions.

Symptoms: White spots, soreness, burning feelings, and trouble swallowing are typical symptoms. In more severe situations, the lesions could reach the throat.

Contributing Factors:

weakened immunity (for example, as a result of immunosuppressive drugs or HIV/AIDS).

usage of antibiotics, which may upset the regular equilibrium of oral microbes.

diabetes, particularly if it is not well managed.

hormonal shifts, such those that occur during pregnancy.

Dry mouth, which lessens the natural defenses provided by saliva.

Usage of drugs that impact the immune system, such as corticosteroids.

Typical in Some Groups:

Infants, the elderly, people with weakened immune systems, and people with underlying medical issues are more likely to have thrush.

Diagnosis: A medical professional's clinical evaluation, frequently verified by a visual study of the distinctive lesions. Swabs may occasionally be collected in order to identify the precise species of Candida through laboratory testing.

Treatment: To address the Candida overgrowth, antifungal drugs like nystatin or clotrimazole are frequently administered. It may be advised to use systemic antifungal drugs for situations that are more severe or persistent.

Preventive actions:

Appropriate dental hygiene procedures, such as routine tongue and tooth brushing.

Washing your mouth after using corticosteroids that you inhaled.

Treating underlying medical issues that could be a factor in thrush.

Avoiding the extended or needless use of antibiotics.

Thrush is usually curable, and problems can be avoided with early treatment. But it can also be a recurrent issue, particularly in those with enduring risk factors. It is essential to comprehend the causes and risk factors of thrush in order to effectively manage and avoid the condition.

Reasons and Danger Elements

The overgrowth of Candida species, especially Candida albicans, in the oral cavity and throat is the cause of thrush, also known as oropharyngeal candidiasis. Thrush can arise from a variety of causes, and some people are more susceptible than others. The following are the main reasons and risk factors for thrush:

1. Reduced Immune Response:

Thrush is more common in those whose immune systems are weakened, such as those with HIV/AIDS, cancer patients, or those on immunosuppressive drugs.

2. Use of Antibiotics:

Antibiotic use has the potential to upset the delicate microbiological balance in the mouth and gastrointestinal system, which promotes the growth of Candida. Thrush is more common in patients treated with broad-spectrum antibiotics.

3. Diabetes:

Uncontrolled diabetes, particularly when combined with elevated blood sugar, creates a favorable environment for Candida to proliferate.

4. Changes in Hormones:

Hormonal changes, such those that happen during pregnancy, might foster an environment where thrush thrives.

5. Parched Mouth:

Thrush risk can be increased by reduced saliva production, which is frequently brought on by situations like dehydration, certain drugs, or medical issues. Saliva contains inherent antifungal qualities that support good dental hygiene.

6. Inhalation of corticosteroids:

Thrush is more common in people who use inhaled corticosteroids for ailments like asthma. After taking these drugs, rinsing the mouth can help lower the risk.

7. Those Who Wear Dentures:

An environment that encourages the growth of Candida and results in thrush can be created by ill-fitting dentures or by denture wearers practicing poor oral care.

8. Age:

Thrush is more common in the elderly and in newborns. The risk in infants is increased by their developing immune systems as well as the presence of candida in the birth canal. Sensitivity is higher in the elderly due to variables including drier oral mucosa and compromised immunity.

9. Smoking:

Smoking can impair immunity and foster an environment in the mouth that is favorable to the growth of fungi.

10. Immunocompromising Situations:

Thrush is more common in patients with immune system-compromising diseases like leukemia and organ transplantation.

11. underlying illnesses:

The risk of thrush can be increased by some medical diseases, such as Sjögren's syndrome, which affects the glands responsible for producing saliva.

To determine who may be more prone to thrush, it is essential to comprehend these causes and risk factors. Thrush and its related consequences can be lessened by treating underlying medical issues, maintaining proper oral hygiene, and adopting preventative steps. Those who are more vulnerable should take extra care to keep their teeth healthy and should get help right once if any signs appear.

Signs and symptoms

The oral cavity and throat are the typical sites of manifestation for thrush, also known as oropharyngeal candidiasis. The following are the most typical signs of thrush:

White lesions are creamy white, cottage cheese-like lesions that can occasionally be found on the tonsils, back of the throat, inside cheeks, and palate. The red, inflammatory tissue beneath these lesions is easily removed.

Pain and Burning Sensations: People who have thrush frequently report pain, burning sensations, or soreness in the mouth and throat regions that are affected.

Difficulty Swallowing: People who have thrush may find it difficult or painful to swallow, and they may have trouble eating or drinking.

Taste Alteration or Loss: People with thrush lesions may experience a change in their taste.

Dry Mouth: Thrush can cause people to experience a dry mouth, which may make them feel as though they need to drink water frequently.

Angulous cheilitis, or cracking and redness at the corners of the mouth, can occasionally result from thrush, particularly in people who wear dentures.

Bad Breath: Halitosis, or bad breath, may be linked to thrush.

It's crucial to remember that symptoms can vary in intensity, and not everyone with thrush will have every symptom on the list. Thrush can occasionally be mild and asymptomatic, particularly in otherwise healthy people.

Similar symptoms, such as white patches on the inside of the cheeks, tongue, and palate, can be seen in infants with thrush. In contrast to adults, it is difficult to remove these patches.

Those receiving chemotherapy or those with HIV/AIDS are examples of people with compromised immune systems who may have more severe and enduring thrush symptoms.

It is best to seek medical attention for a proper diagnosis and appropriate treatment if someone feels they may have thrush, especially if they show the typical white lesions or have discomfort in the mouth. Antifungal drugs are usually used in treatment to target the Candida overgrowth and reduce symptoms.

Identification and Medical Assessment

Thrush, also known as oropharyngeal candidiasis, is diagnosed mainly through clinical evaluation by a medical practitioner. The diagnosis and medical assessment of thrush usually involve the following steps:

CHAPTER TWO

Clinical Assessment:

An oral health professional, usually a dentist, will perform a comprehensive examination of the oral cavity. They will be on the lookout for telltale symptoms of thrush, such as creamy white lesions on the palate, inner cheeks, tongue, and other oral mucosa areas.

Health Background:

Gathering a complete medical history is vital. The healthcare professional will inquire about the patient's overall health, any underlying medical issues, drugs being taken, recent antibiotic use, and other pertinent circumstances.

Visual Inspection:

The healthcare provider will visually inspect the lesions to assess their appearance, location, and distribution. The characteristic cottage cheese-like appearance of the lesions is often indicative of thrush.

Swab and Culture:

In some cases, a swab may be taken from the affected areas to collect samples for laboratory testing. These samples can be cultured to identify the specific Candida species responsible for the infection.

Microscopic Examination:

Microscopic examination of the swab samples may be performed to confirm the presence of Candida yeast cells and hyphae.

Underlying Conditions:

The healthcare provider may explore underlying illnesses or risk factors that could contribute to the development of thrush, such as immunosuppression, diabetes, or usage of drugs that influence the immune system.

Systemic Evaluation:

In cases when thrush is severe or recurrent, and especially if there are concerns about systemic involvement, a more extensive evaluation of the patient's overall health may be done.

Testing for Underlying Conditions:

If an underlying problem is detected, more testing or referrals to experts may be advised to address and manage the contributing causes.

It's crucial for anyone having symptoms suggestive of thrush, such as the presence of white sores in the mouth or discomfort, to seek quick medical assistance. A quick and precise diagnosis allows for optimal therapy with antifungal drugs, such as clotrimazole or nystatin, which are usually administered to attack the Candida overgrowth.

In circumstances where thrush is persistent or recurrent, a full medical assessment may be necessary to detect and manage any underlying health conditions contributing to the illness. Regular follow-up with the healthcare practitioner is crucial to monitor the response to treatment and manage any contributing factors.

The treatment of thrush, or oropharyngeal candidiasis, often requires antifungal drugs to target the overgrowth of Candida species. The choice of treatment relies on the severity of the illness, underlying health issues, and the specific circumstances of the individual. Here are common treatment techniques for thrush:

Topical Antifungals:

Nystatin: A routinely used antifungal drug for oral thrush. It is available in several forms, including oral suspensions or lozenges. Nystatin is swished about the lips and then swallowed or administered topically to the afflicted areas.

Another antifungal medication that comes in lozenges is clotrimazole. It offers targeted therapy and dissolves in the tongue.

Antifungals in the System:

Fluconazole: Systemic antifungal drugs such as fluconazole may be recommended in cases of more severe or persistent thrush, or in situations when topical therapies are ineffective. This oral drug works throughout the body to prevent Candida from growing.

Maintenance of Dentures:

If wearing dentures is linked to thrush, cleaning and maintaining denture hygiene is essential. People should clean their dentures on a regular basis and adhere to their healthcare provider's advice on how to treat thrush when wearing dentures.

Duration of Treatment:

Depending on the severity of the infection and the patient's reaction to antifungal therapy, the length of the treatment may change. Even if symptoms subside before the recommended drug course is completed, it is still necessary to take the entire advised course of action.

Handling Contextual Factors:

Long-term prevention of thrush requires addressing and treating underlying medical issues like diabetes or immunosuppression that contribute to the disease. In order to effectively manage underlying diseases, various healthcare specialists may need to collaborate.

Maintaining Good Dental Hygiene

Maintaining proper dental care is essential to avoiding thrush recurrence. Maintaining oral health involves brushing your teeth, tongue, and gums on a regular basis and using an antimicrobial mouthwash as directed by your doctor.

Continuation Care:

It's important to follow up with the doctor on a regular basis to discuss any concerns or inquiries, evaluate how the treatment is working, and track the progress of the symptoms.

Preventive actions:

People who are susceptible to recurrent thrush should take precautions, such as practicing good oral hygiene, abstaining from overusing antibiotics, taking care of any underlying medical issues, and following recommended treatment regimens.

It's critical that patients heed the advice of their medical professional and report any lingering or worsening symptoms both during and after therapy. When thrush is linked to underlying medical diseases or risk factors, a complete management strategy could be required. In order to obtain the best results, healthcare providers are essential in customizing treatment regimens to meet the needs of each patient and addressing any relevant factors.

Oropharyngeal candidiasis, or thrush, can be prevented by practicing good oral hygiene, taking care of any underlying medical issues, and reducing risk factors that could lead to Candida overgrowth. The following are thrush preventative measures:

Maintaining Good Dental Hygiene

Use fluoride toothpaste to routinely brush your teeth, tongue, and gums.

To clean in between teeth, use dental floss or an interdental brush.

Use an antiseptic mouthwash to rinse your mouth as directed by your healthcare provider.

Maintenance of Dentures:

Make sure your dentures fit well and are cleaned on a regular basis if you wear them.

Every day, take out and wash your dentures to avoid Candida colonization.

Steer clear of unnecessary antibiotics:

Antibiotics should only be taken as directed by medical professionals.

Talk about the possible effects of antibiotics on the balance of Candida and the oral microbiome with the healthcare provider.

Handling Concomitant Medical Conditions:

Effectively treat illnesses like diabetes or HIV/AIDS that can compromise immunity.

Seek routine medical attention and adhere to the recommended course of treatment for any underlying medical conditions.

Steer clear of Needless Corticosteroids:

To lower the risk of thrush when using inhaled corticosteroids, thoroughly rinse your mouth after each use.

A nutritious diet

Keep your diet nutrient-rich and well-balanced to support immune system and general health.

Restrict your intake of sweetened foods and drinks because they can exacerbate Candida overgrowth.

Maintain Hydration:

Water consumption should be sufficient to avoid dry mouth, since decreased salivary flow can raise the risk of thrush.

Frequent dental examinations:

Plan for routine dental cleanings and examinations to keep an eye on your oral health and take quick action to address any issues.

Quick Resolution of Oral Infections:

If you see any symptoms of an oral infection, such as soreness or white lesions, get medical help right once.

Maintain a Healthy Lifestyle:

Engage in regular exercise to support overall health.

Avoid smoking, as smoking affects the immune system and contributes to oral health problems.

Education and Awareness:

Stay informed about the risk factors and symptoms of thrush.

Educate individuals at higher risk, such as those with weakened immune systems, about preventive measures.

Consider Probiotics:

Probiotics may help maintain a healthy balance of microorganisms in the gut and potentially reduce the risk of Candida overgrowth.

It's important to tailor preventive measures to individual health needs and risk factors. Individuals with specific risk factors or medical conditions may benefit from personalized advice from healthcare professionals. Regular communication with healthcare providers and a proactive approach to oral health contribute to effective prevention and early intervention in case of any concerns.

CHAPTER THREE

Candida and Systemic Health

Candida, the yeast responsible for thrush (oropharyngeal candidiasis), is a part of the normal microbiota in the human body, typically residing in the gastrointestinal tract and mucous membranes. While Candida is generally harmless in small amounts, overgrowth or an imbalance in the microbial community can lead to infections, including thrush. Beyond the localized effects in the oral cavity, Candida overgrowth has been associated with systemic health implications in certain circumstances. Here are some considerations related to Candida and systemic health:

Immune System Interaction:

Individuals with weakened immune systems, such as those with HIV/AIDS or undergoing chemotherapy, are more susceptible to Candida overgrowth and systemic infections. Candida can exploit impaired immune responses, leading to invasive infections and affecting various organs.

Systemic Candidiasis:

In severe circumstances, Candida can enter the bloodstream and produce systemic candidiasis. This syndrome may lead to disseminated infections affecting organs such as the liver, spleen, kidneys, and heart. Systemic candidiasis is a significant medical illness that demands immediate and strong treatment.

Underlying Health Conditions:

Numerous medical issues, including as autoimmune illnesses, chronic inflammatory ailments, and gastrointestinal disorders have been linked to Candida overgrowth. Although the exact nature of this relationship is still unknown, some evidence indicates that changes to the gut microbiota, such as an overabundance of Candida, may have an impact on overall health.

Gut-Brain Axis:

The gut microbiota, including Candida, plays a function in the gut-brain axis, a bidirectional communication pathway between the gut and the central neurological system. Imbalances in the gut microbiota, particularly Candida overgrowth, have been implicated in illnesses such as irritable bowel syndrome (IBS) and mental disorders.

Chronic Inflammation:

Persistent Candida overgrowth may contribute to chronic inflammation, potentially compromising systemic health. Chronic inflammation is related with several health issues, including cardiovascular disease and metabolic diseases.

Immune Modulation:

Candida can affect the host immune response, altering immune cells and their actions. This immune modification may have systemic implications beyond the site of infection.

Risk in Immunocompetent Individuals:

In immunocompetent individuals, systemic consequences of Candida are infrequent. However, protracted or recurrent cases of localized infections, such as thrush, may prompt inquiry into potential underlying problems impacting systemic health.

It's crucial to note that while Candida overgrowth has been examined in relation to systemic health, the exact nature of these relationships and the involvement of Candida in various illnesses are areas of continuing research. Additionally, the vast majority of persons with localized thrush do not develop systemic symptoms.

A comprehensive strategy that includes immunological support, lifestyle changes, and the care of underlying medical disorders may be necessary to address systemic health issues associated with Candida. Individuals suffering symptoms suggestive of systemic candidiasis or those with concerns about the influence of Candida on their health should seek help from healthcare specialists for appropriate examination and management.

DIY Solutions & Self-Treatment

While the main method of treating thrush is medical intervention, which includes antifungal drugs given by medical professionals, there are several at-home cures and self-care practices that people can do to support the treatment and lessen symptoms. It's crucial to remember that these remedies are only meant to be used in addition to medical guidance and recommended therapies. Here are some thrush home cures and self-care advice:

Sustain Proper Dental Hygiene:

Use fluoride toothpaste to routinely brush your teeth, tongue, and gums.

To clean in between teeth, use dental floss or an interdental brush.

Use an antiseptic mouthwash to rinse your mouth as directed by your healthcare provider.

Warm Seawater Rinse:

Gargling with warm seawater can help reduce thrush-related discomfort. Gargle with a solution made up of one teaspoon salt and warm water.

Probiotics:

Foods and supplements high in probiotics may aid in reestablishing the oral microbiome's equilibrium. Lactobacillus and other helpful bacteria are found in probiotics, which may be advantageous.

Yogurt

Eating plain, unsweetened yogurt that has live cultures in it may help keep the bacteria in the mouth and stomach in a healthy balance.

Limit Your Sugar Consumption:

Cut back on sugar-filled foods and drinks because these can encourage the overgrowth of Candida. A sugar-free or low-sugar diet could be helpful.

Coconut Oil:

Some people get relief by oil pulling, or swishing coconut oil around in their mouths. The antifungal effects of coconut oil are possible. After swishing, spit the oil out rather than swallowing it.

Garlic

It is well known that garlic may have antifungal effects. Garlic pills or adding fresh garlic to the diet are options to think about. However, before using supplements containing garlic, speak with a medical expert.

Mild Mouth Rinses:

Use diluted hydrogen peroxide or a weak solution of baking soda and water to rinse the mouth (as directed by the product). These remedies might improve dental health by lessening mouth acidity.

Maintain Hydration:

Water consumption should be sufficient to avoid dry mouth, since decreased salivary flow might raise the risk of thrush.

Steer clear of alcohol and tobacco:

An increased risk of oral health issues can be attributed to smoking and binge drinking. Steer clear of these drugs, if possible.

Dietary Adjustments:

Think about using a diet that enhances immune system and general wellness. Incorporate foods high in nutrients to support optimum health.

Frequent dental examinations:

Plan for routine dental cleanings and examinations to keep an eye on your oral health and take quick action to address any issues.

Before attempting any home treatments, it is imperative to speak with a healthcare provider, particularly in cases where underlying medical issues are present or if self-care measures are ineffective in treating the thrush. These actions don't replace recommended medical treatments, even though they might reduce symptoms. It is imperative to seek urgent medical attention for an appropriate diagnosis and action if symptoms worsen or do not improve with home cures.

In summary, thrush, also known as oropharyngeal candidiasis, is a fungal infection that affects the throat and oral cavity and is typically caused by the species Candida albicans. Thrush is typically localized, but it can also affect the entire body, particularly in those with compromised immune systems or underlying medical issues. These are the main ideas to wrap up the subject:

Reasons and Danger Factors:

Candida yeast overgrowth, which is the cause of thrush, is frequently brought on by conditions like diabetes, dry mouth, antibiotic use, compromised immunity, and hormonal changes.

Signs:

Thrush is characterized by white, cottage cheese-like lesions on the tongue, inner cheeks, and other oral mucosa; the lesions are accompanied by pain, burning, and trouble swallowing.

Clinical examination, medical history, and, in certain situations, swab samples for laboratory testing to identify the particular species of Candida are all part of the diagnosis process.

Therapy:

Antifungal drugs, fluconazole, nystatin, and clotrimazole being examples of topical and systemic treatments, are frequently used with the goal of suppressing the overgrowth of Candida.

Preventive actions:

Preventive approaches encompass the following: regulating lifestyle variables, preventing needless antibiotic use, treating underlying medical disorders, and practicing good oral hygiene.

DIY Solutions & Self-Treatment:

Warm saltwater gargles, probiotics, yogurt, coconut oil, and dietary adjustments are examples of supportive interventions that can be used at home. Nonetheless, these need to supplement medical advice and approved therapies, not take their place.

Systemic Health Consequences:

Though limited, Candida overgrowth in thrush can affect the entire body, especially in those with weakened immune systems. Systemic candidiasis is a serious illness that needs to be treated right away.

Frequent observation and follow-up:

Monitoring oral health, treating issues, and controlling any underlying diseases all depend on routine dental checkups and follow-up visits with medical professionals.

People who have thrush symptoms or who are at danger of getting it again should get medical help very away. If the right treatments are used, thrush is usually curable, and prevention is key to lowering the chance of recurrence. Through comprehension of the etiology, manifestations, and therapeutic approaches of thrush, people can proactively enhance their oral health and general welfare.

THE END